Harry's Big Day at the dentist

BY RICHARD SCHMIDT

Second Edition 2013

Harry's Big Day *at the dentist*
By Richard Schmidt

Copyright © 2013 Richard Schmidt

All rights reserved. This book or any portion thereof may not be reproduced or used in any manner whatsoever without the express written permission of the publisher except for the use of brief quotations in a book review.

Illustrations by digitalstudio/Bigstock.com

Printed in te United States

ackowledgements

the people who have had the greatest impact on my life and encouraged me to dream:

My mother Rebecca Giaquinta, who has given me the inspiration and encouragement to write this book.

My stepfather Robert Giaquinta DDS, who I have learned so much from.

Hysson Monia, who was critical in helping provide content and structure, as well as amazing support for my efforts.

All my teachers, colleagues and patients past and present; your contribution to my life and subsequently this book have been immense.

Finally I want to thank you, the reader, for recognizing that good dental health is essential to healthier living and having the ambition and drive to want to fulfill your potential. I hope that this may inspire you to help others as well. Spread the word.

Thank you,

Richard Schmidt

Harry's Big Day at the dentist

"Good morning Harry, it's time to wake up." Harry's mother said as she entered his bedroom. Harry wasn't a little boy anymore. After all, he is getting ready to start kindergarten like all big boys do.

"I'm a big boy," Harry said to his mother with a big grin. "Soon I'll be going to school," he continued.

"That's right and do you know what big boys have to do before they can start school?" his mother asked.

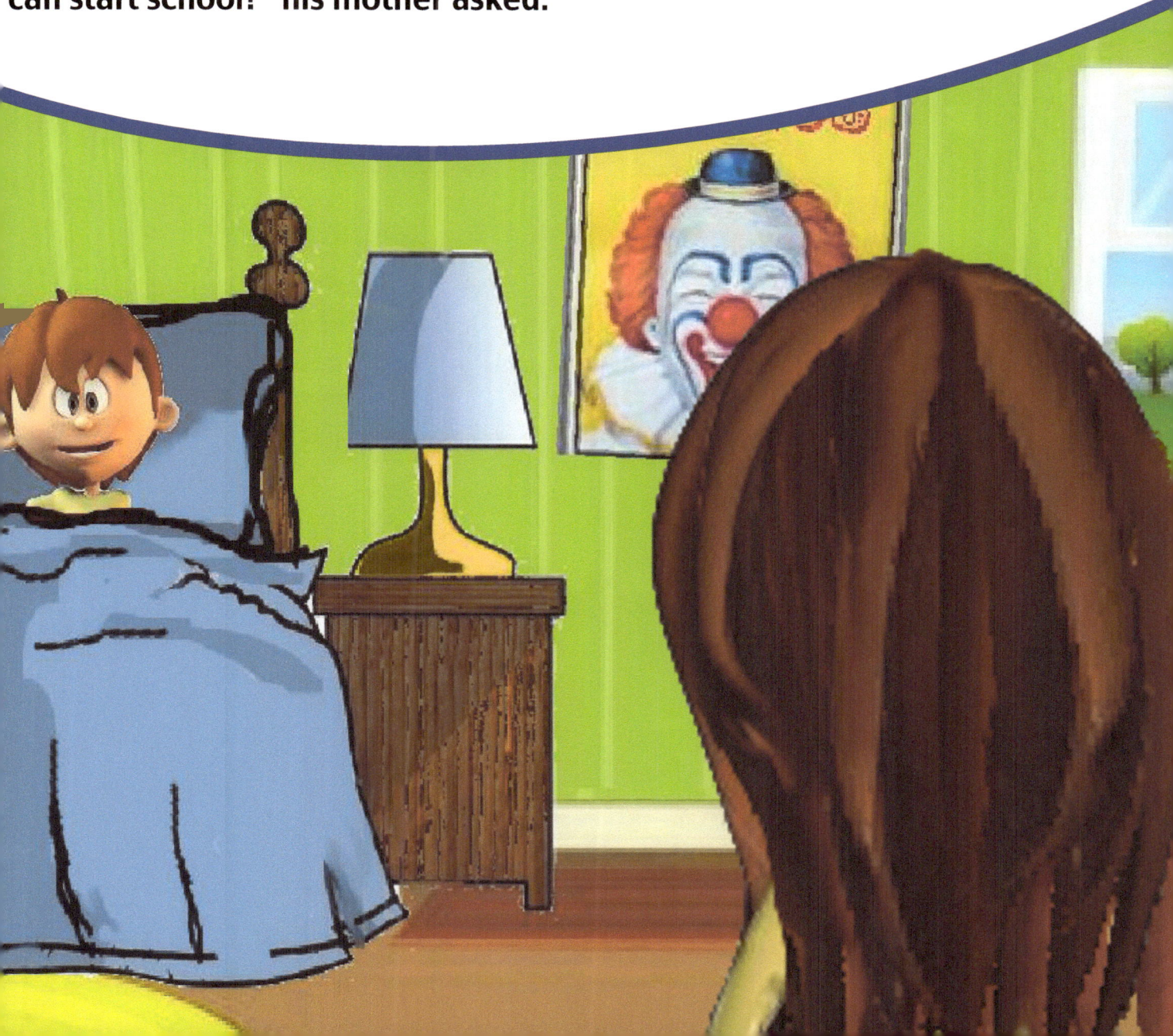

"Um, tie my shoes?" Answered Harry.

"Well ahh yes, yes, but also great to go to the dentist for teeth counted and shined.

"Why have told and shined?" He asked.

"Because the school only allows children with brighter teeth in class. It is therefore very important to always keep them bright and shiny. We have a dentist appointment this afternoon and he will make sure they are bright enough to you go to school. "her mother replied.

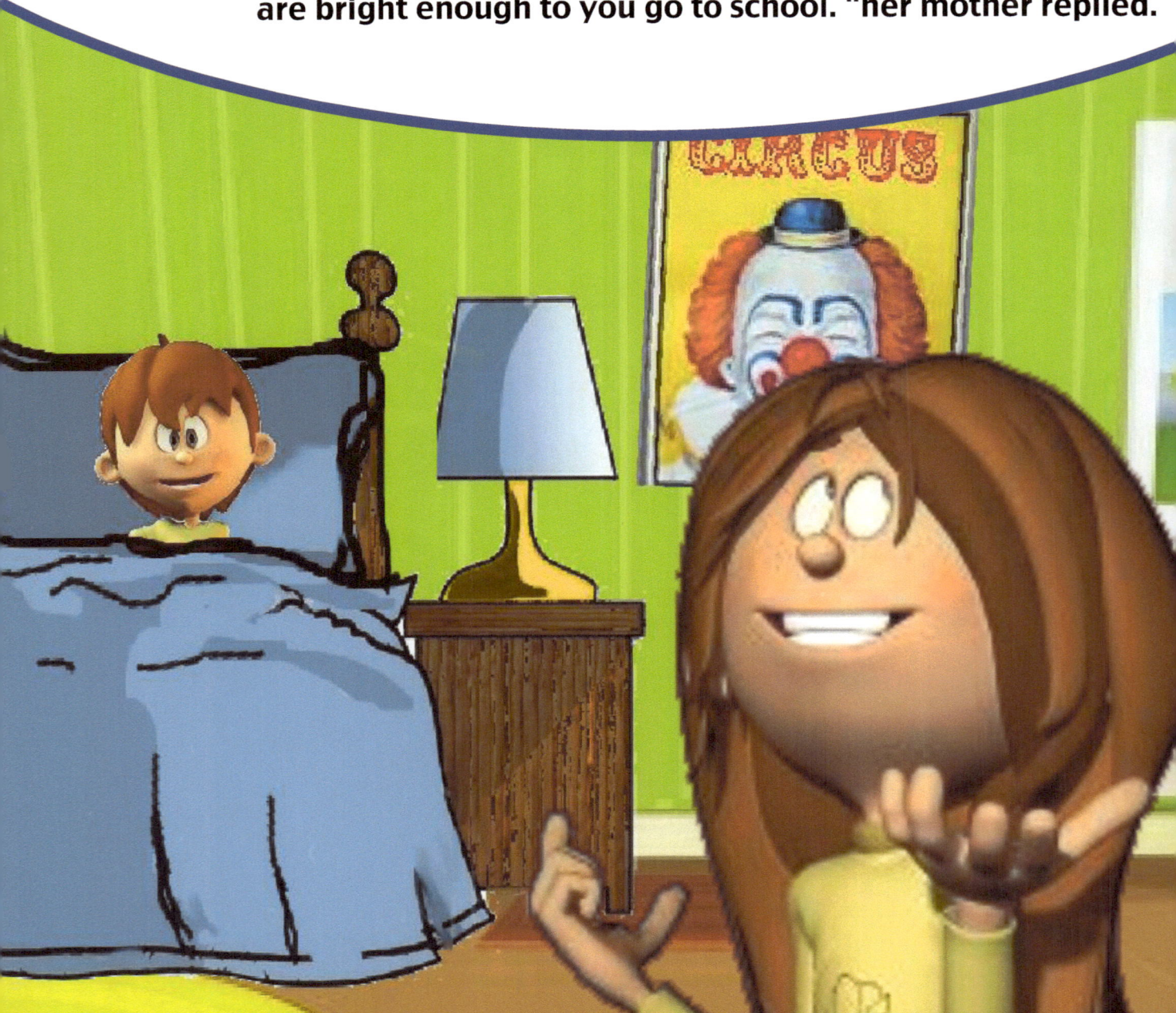

So Harry and his mother got dressed and went to the city to see the dentist. Harry began to wonder if his teeth were going to be bright enough for school, and what if the other children's teeth were brighter than his. "Mom, what if my teeth are not bright enough for school?" Harry asked with a worried look

"That's why we go to the dentist dear. He will ensure that they are and it will show you how to keep them that way." his mother replied.

As they turned the corner Harry's mother pointed to a large brick building and said, "Harry look at your new school."

"Wow, it's huge!" Harry shouted: "I hope you do not get lost inside there."

"Do not worry, no," his mother said reassuringly.

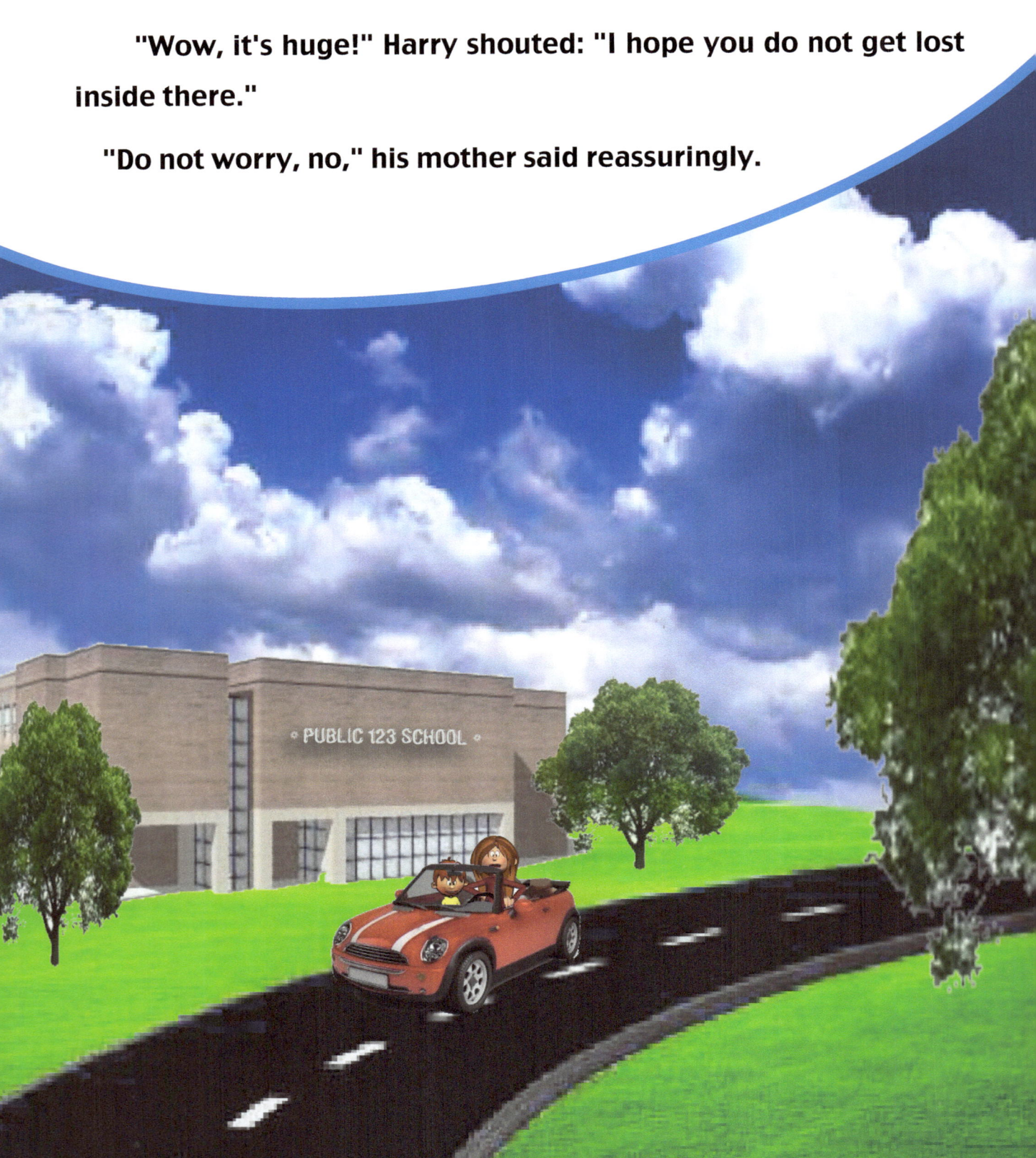

"Well, here we are, we made it just in time." his mother said as they hurried into the office.

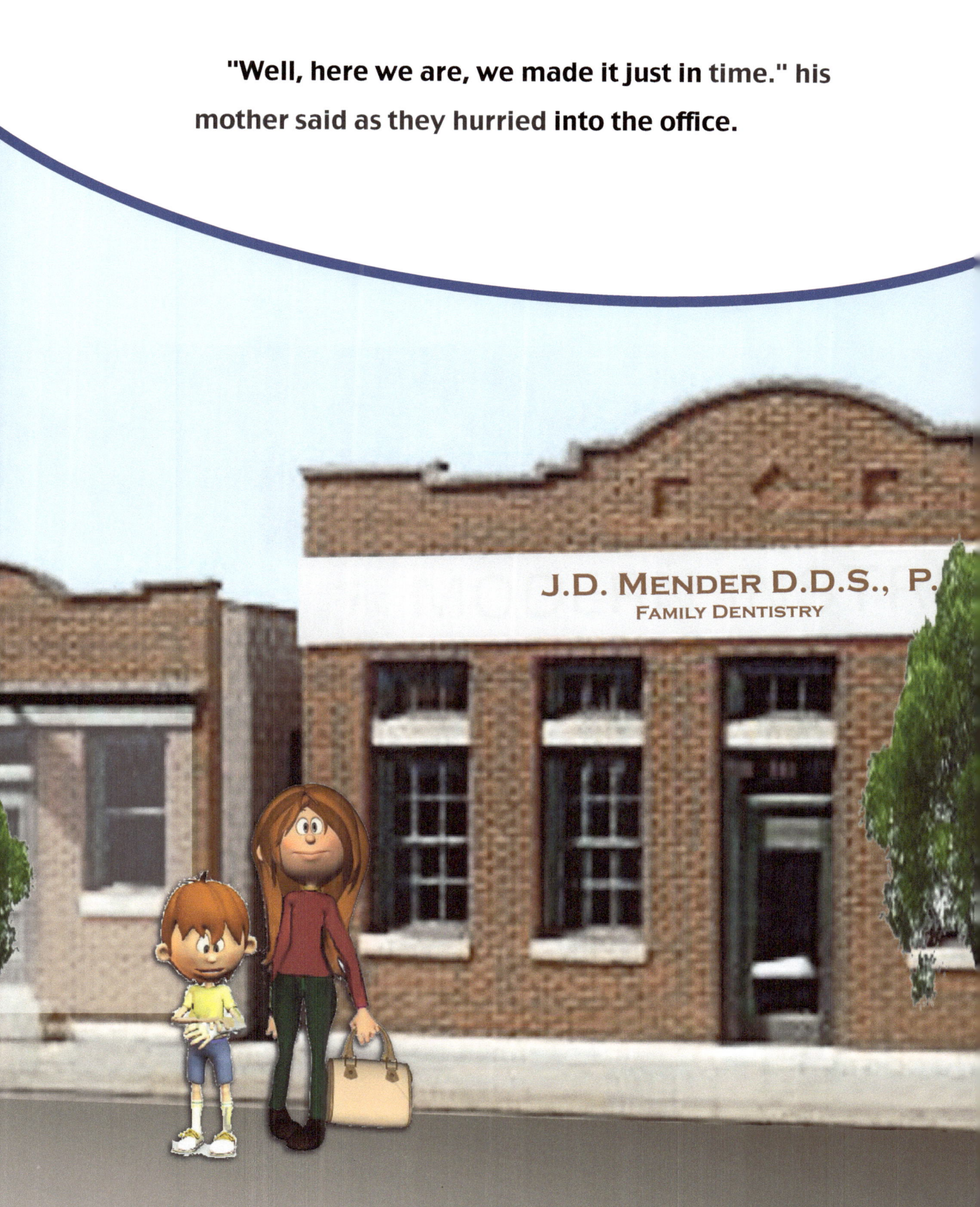

Harry's mother told the woman at the desk that they were there for Harry's 1pm appointment.

"Have a seat and I will tell the Doctor you are here," the receptionist replied.

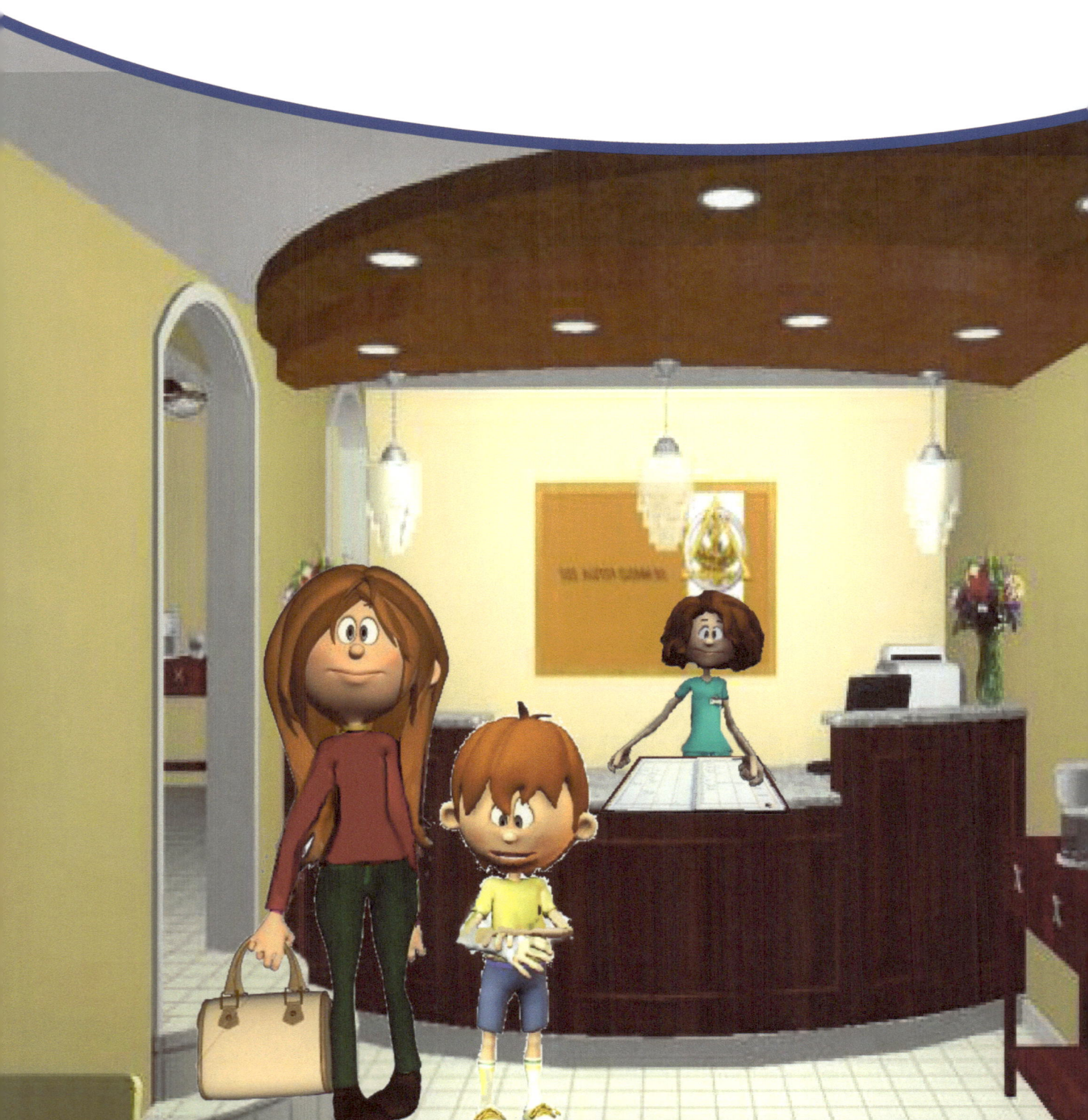

"Hello Harry, I see you are here for a check-up." the dentist said as he entered the room

"Yes Doctor, it's for school, I'm a big boy now," Harry said with a smile.

"You certainly are, but before we get started counting and shining your teeth we will need to take some special pictures called x-rays of your teeth. Shall we get started?" the dentist asked.

"Yes sir," Harry answered.

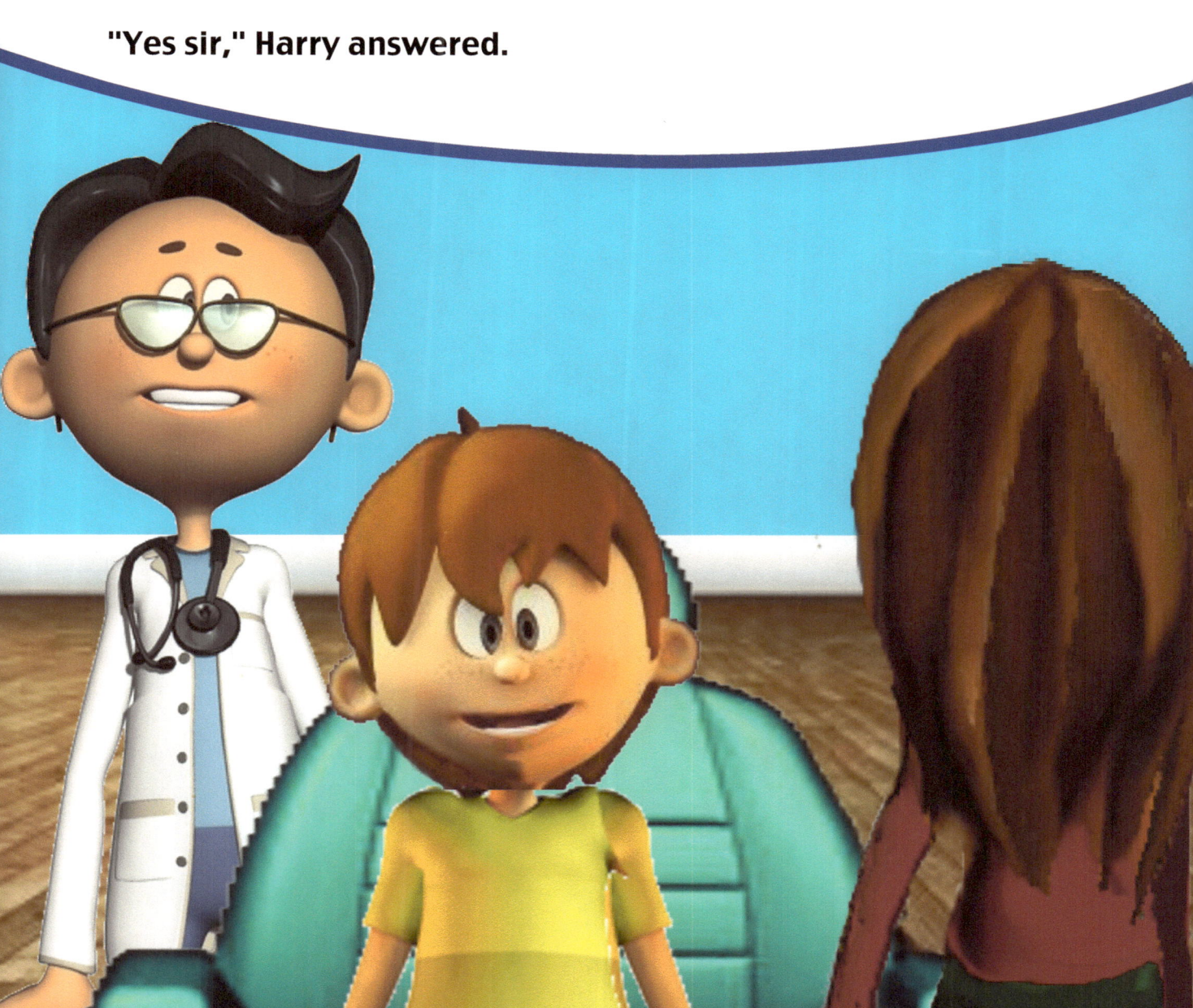

The dental assistant came in and said she had to put a heavy blanket on Harry so the special camera will only takes pictures of his teeth. Then she moved a big camera over to his face and told him to stay very still. Harry did as he was told, because hedidn't want to mess up the picture. The camera made a BUZZZZ noise as she pressed the button and suddenly a picture of Harry's teeth appeared on the screen.

"That's Cool," Harry shouted.

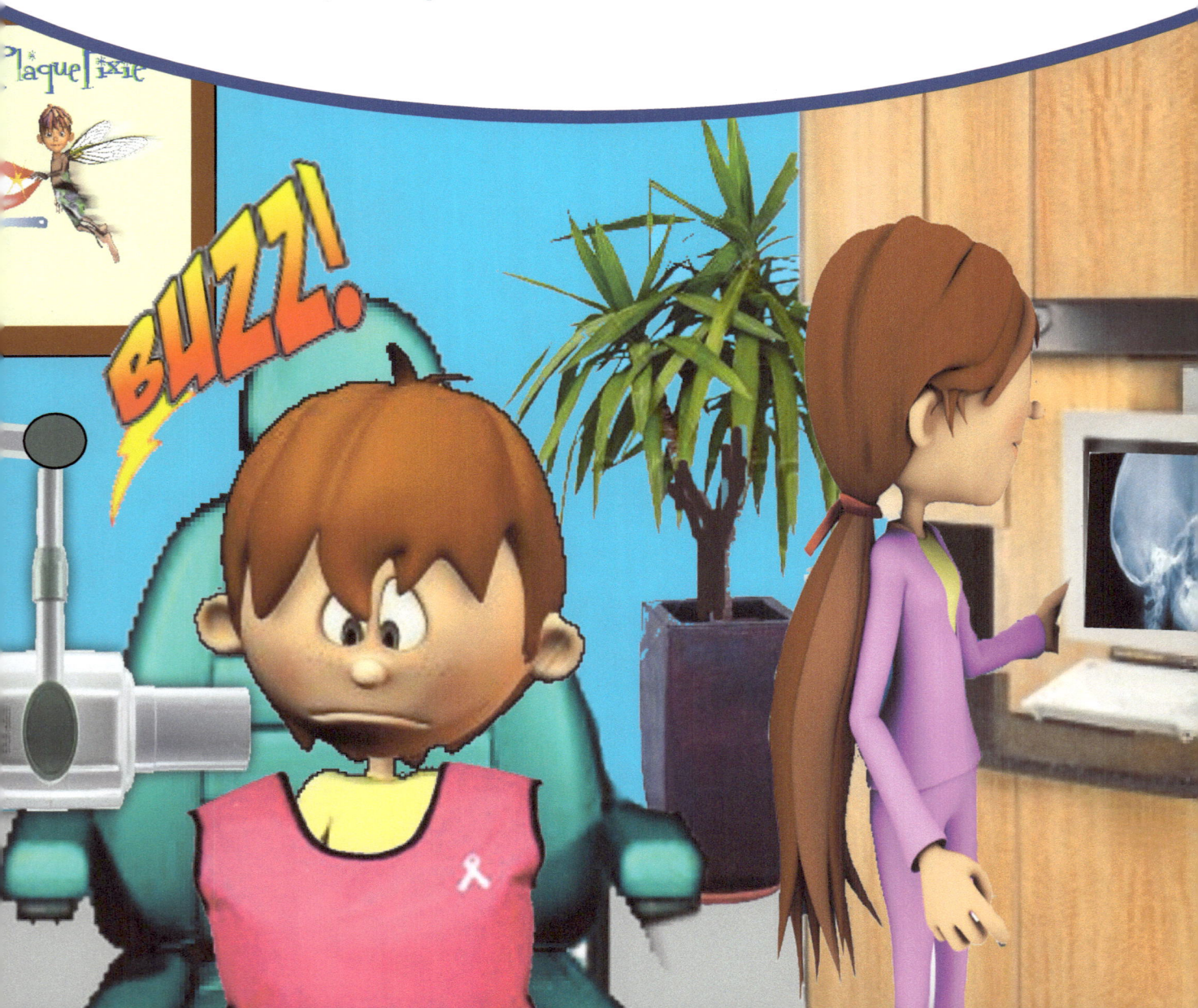

The dentist came back in said x-rays looked good. Then he picked up a special hook shaped counter and little mirror for the check-up. Harry asked why he needed those things and he said to see all the way in the back. The he started counting "1, 2, 3..... 20..... WOW!, did you know that you have 20 teeth?" the dentist asked.

"No,"Harry asked, "is that too many?"

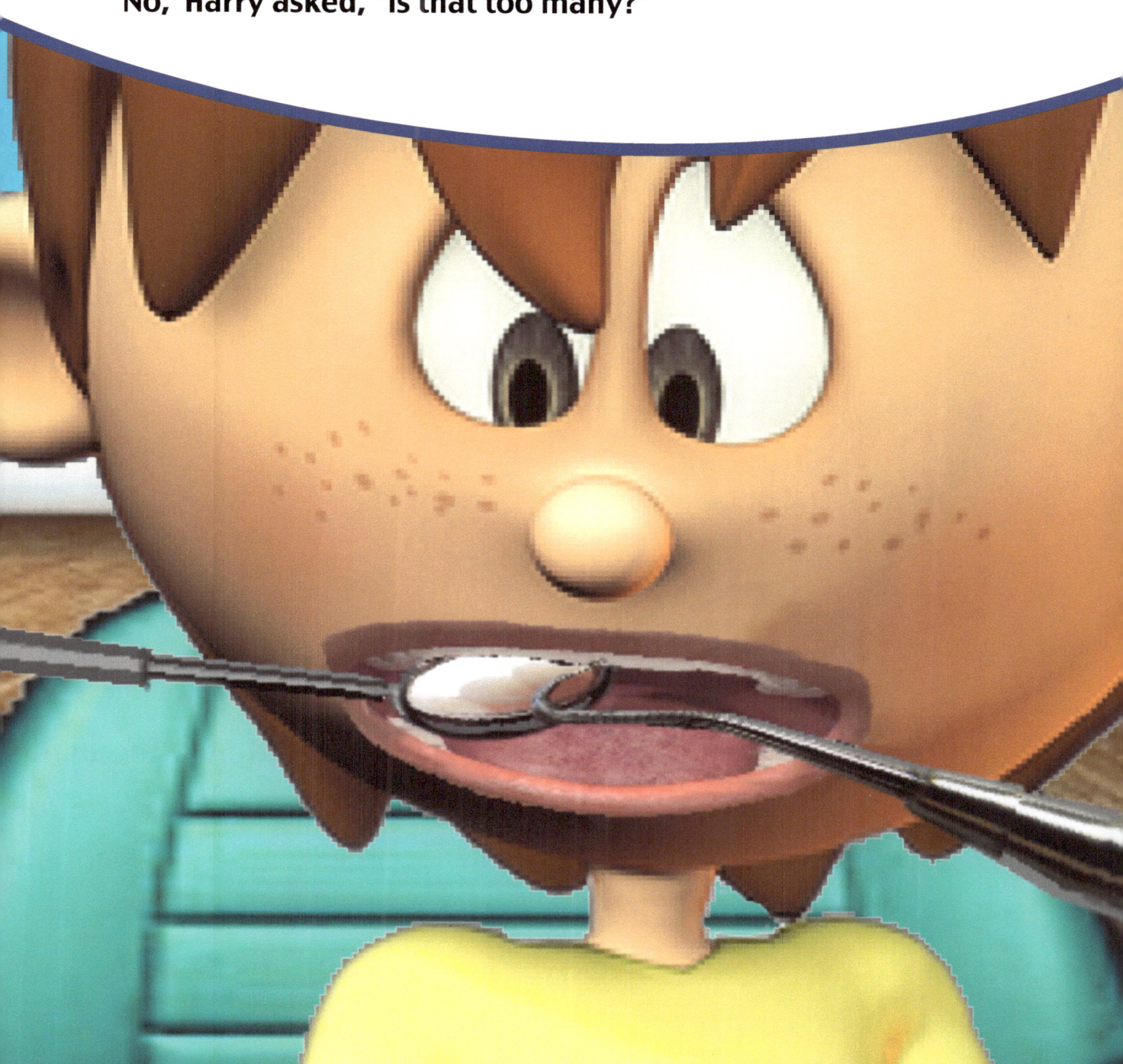

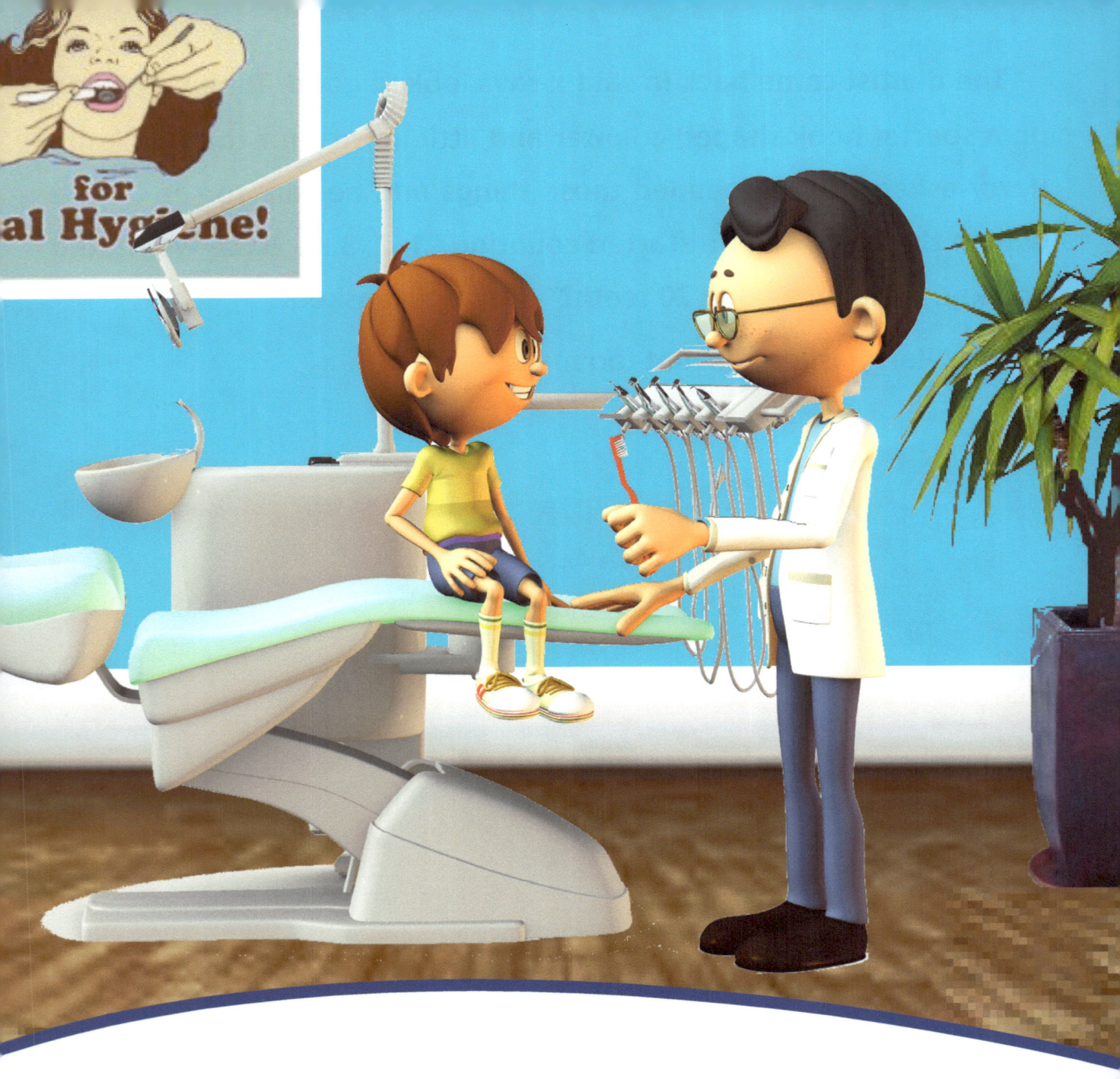

"Nope, it is just the right amount for 5 year old boy, the dentist replied. Because when you turn 6 years old, you will start to get your #rst permanent teeth. They are called 6 year molars and they will come in right behind the ones you already have. Now it's time to to make your teeth shiny and bright so you will be certain to get into class." he continued.

Then the dentist used an electric toothbrush to make Harry's teeth shiny and bright for his first day at school. At first Harry thought it would hurt, but he couldn't stop laughing because it tickled so much and he really liked the bubblegum flavored toothpaste they used. Harry was happy to learn that he could use any flavor toothpaste as long as it had fluoride in it.

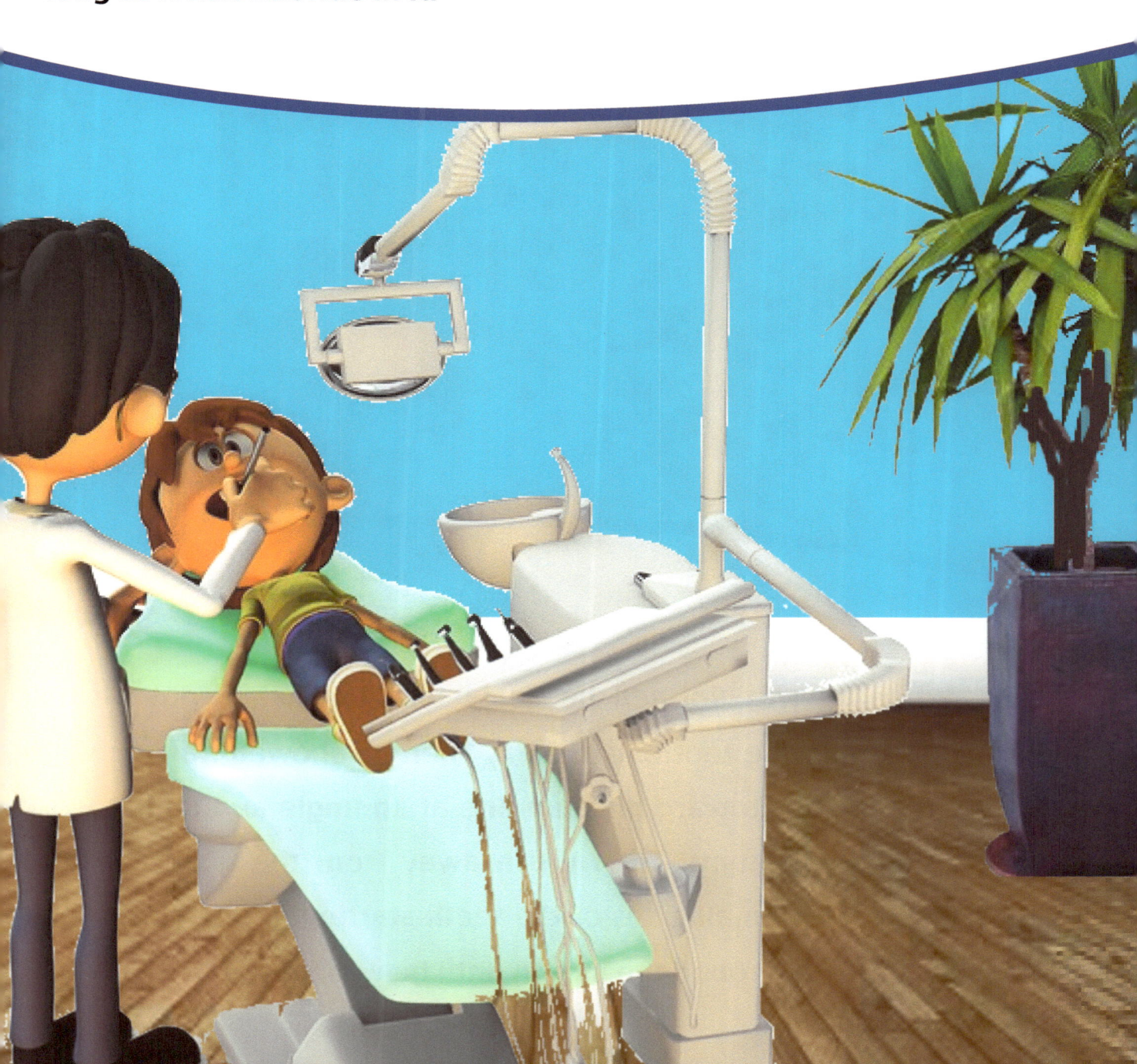

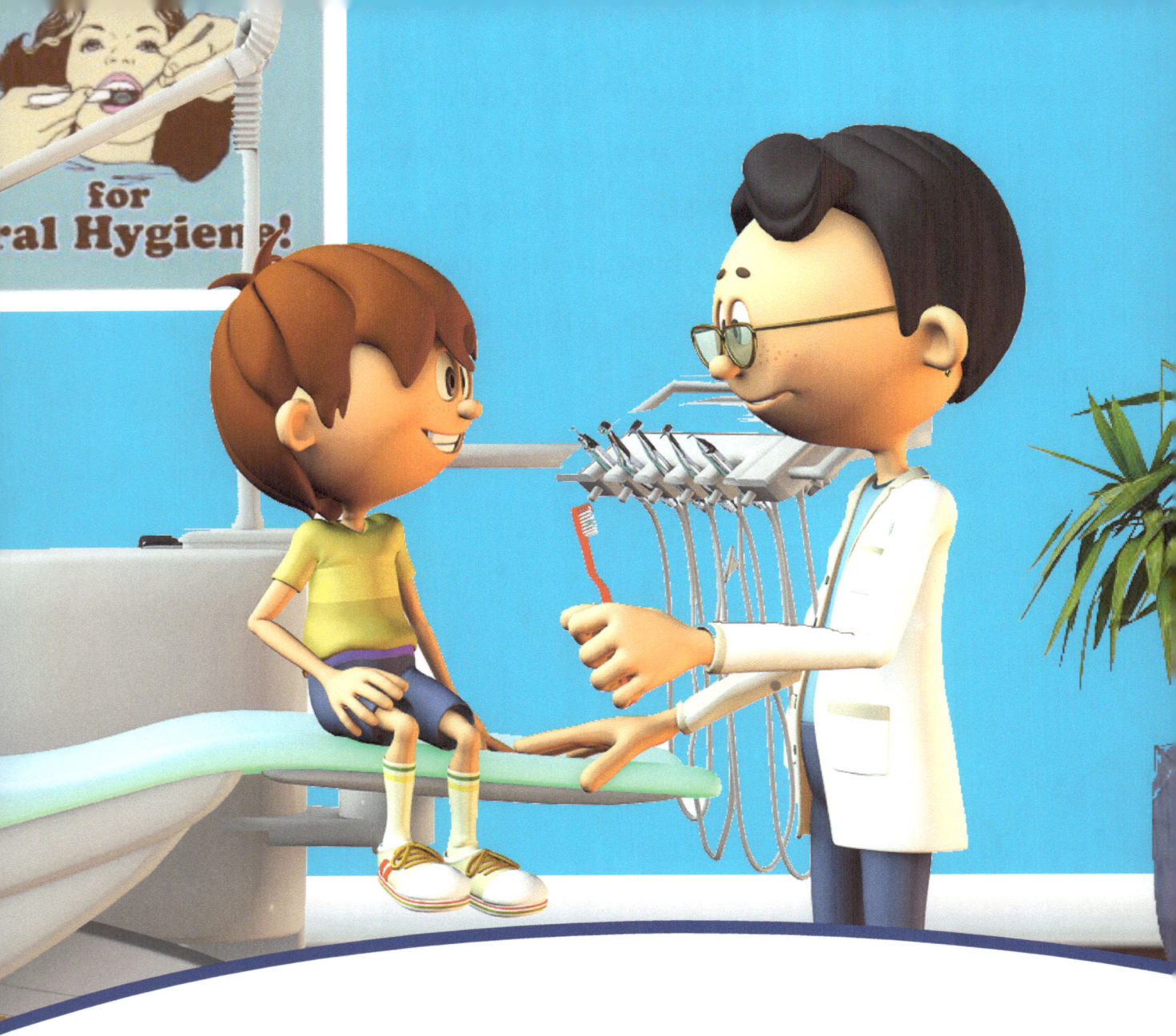

When he was finished he got a toothbrush and put a small amount of fluoride toothpaste on it. Then he showed Harry how to point the bristles toward his gum line at an angle and gently work them under the gums. Then brush away from the gums. He told Harry to do this on all sides of the teeth starting in one corner and working his way around the mouth until he was finished.

Then the dentist handed Harry the toothbrush and told Harry to show him what he just learned.

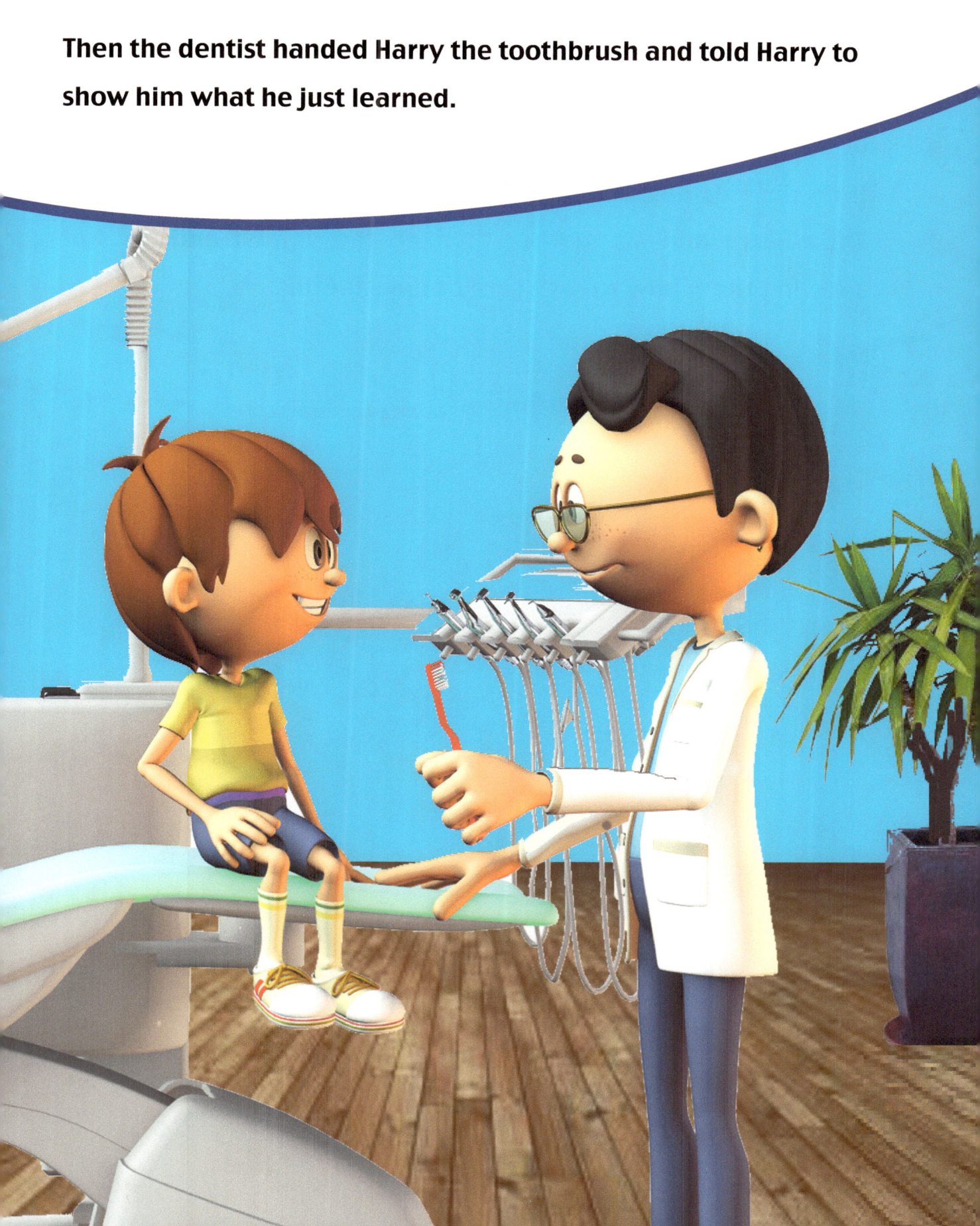

Harry took the toothbrush, and just as the dentist showed him, brushed his teeth starting on the upper right in the back and working his way around to the other side. The dentist told them that if he did this day and night his teeth would stay bright and shiny. Then Harry and his mother thanked the dentist and his staff for showing them how to take care of their teeth.

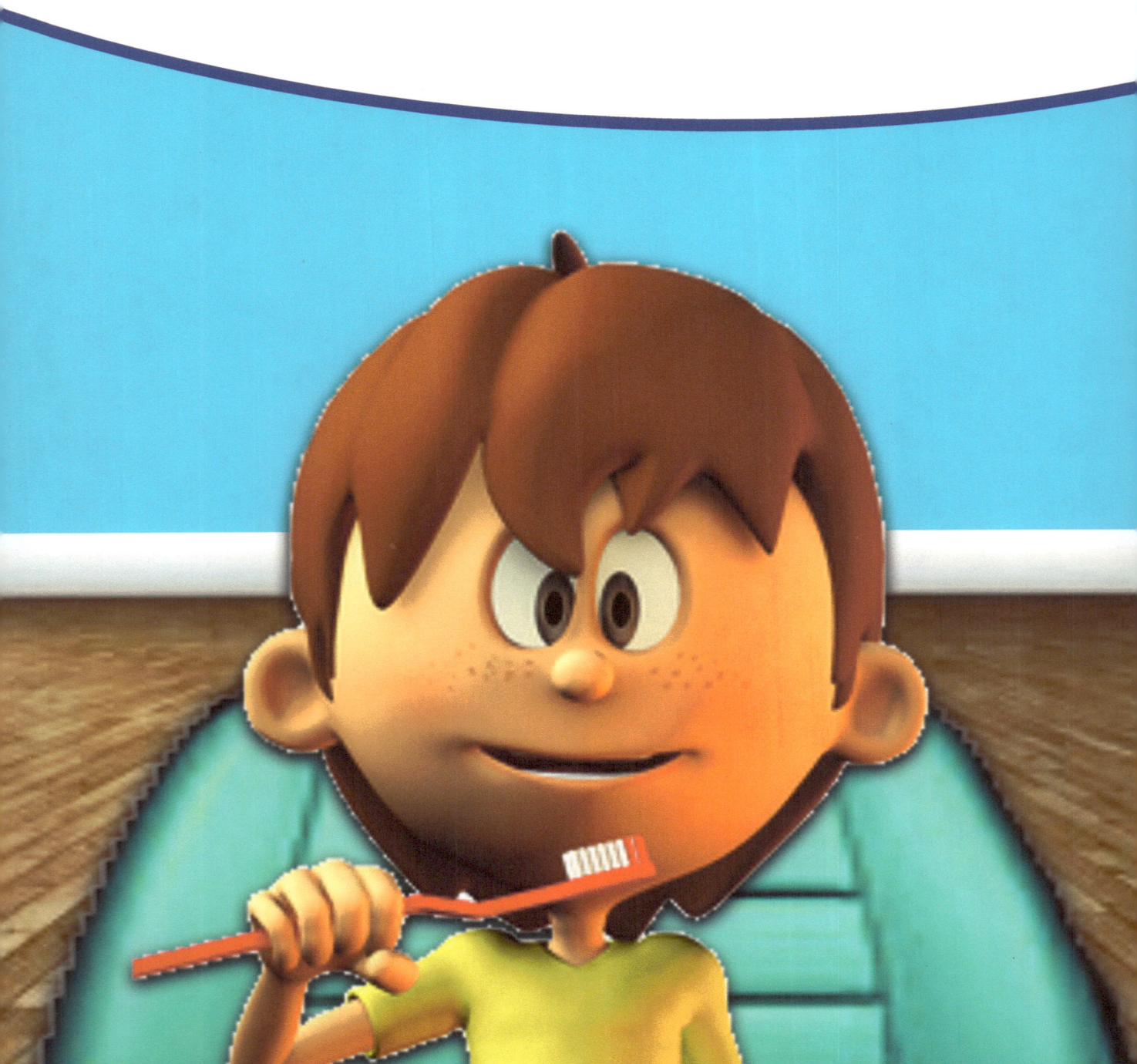

Harry was so excited about his shiny teeth he looked at them all the way home.

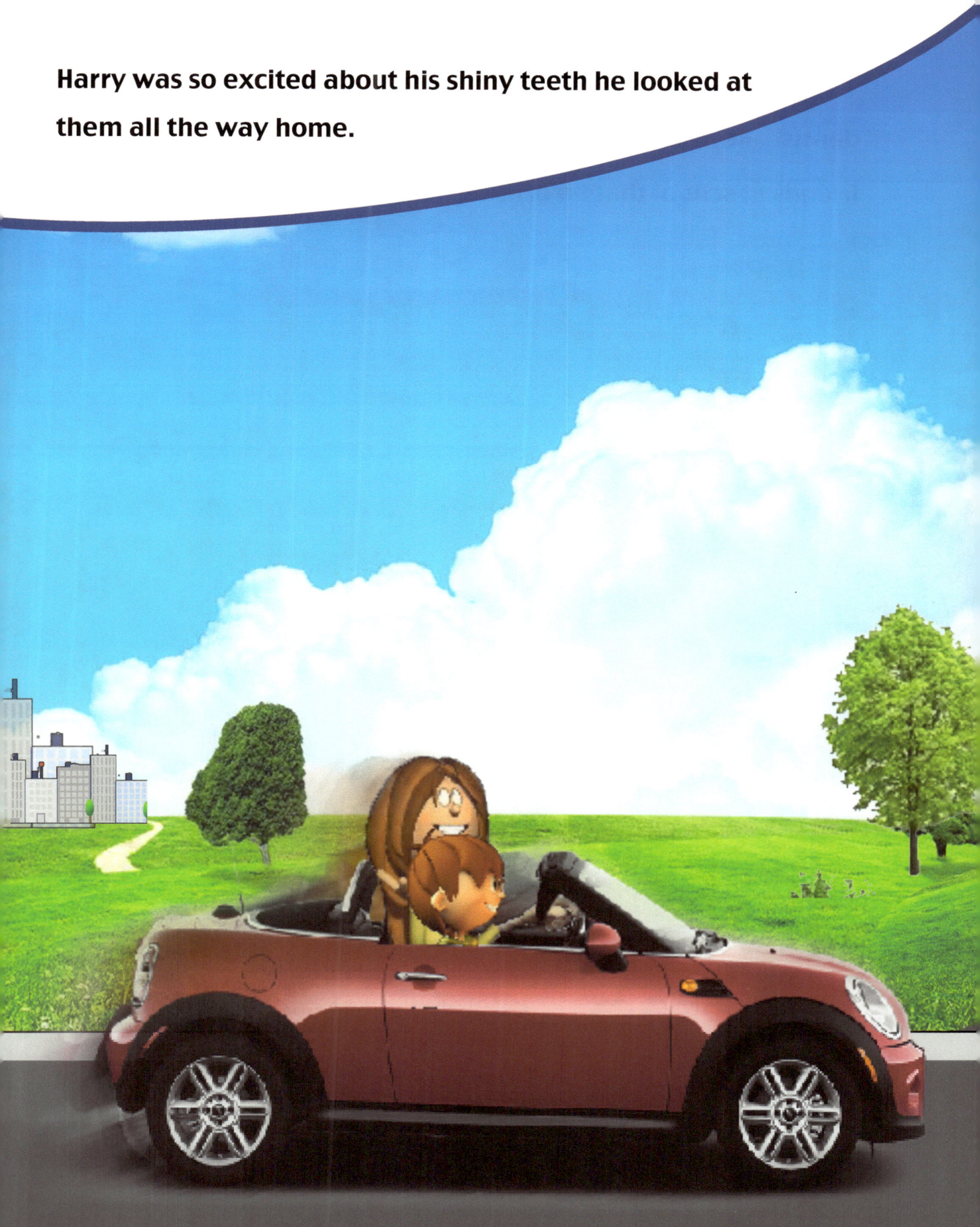

Harry kept his teeth shiny and clean ever since that day at the dentist. He was so excited to show off his shiny teeth to his new friends at school that he brushed **DAY...**

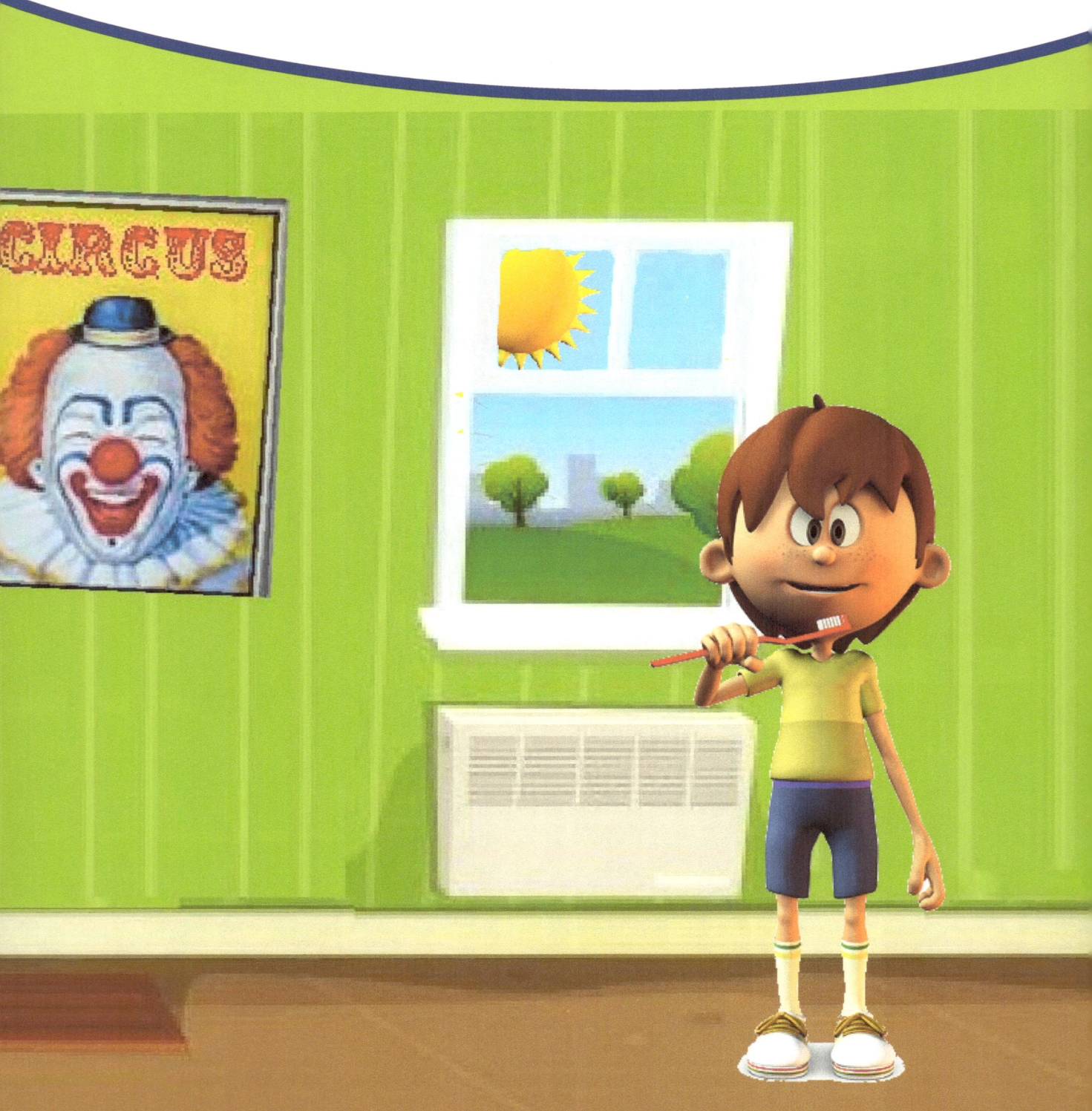

...and **NIGHT.**

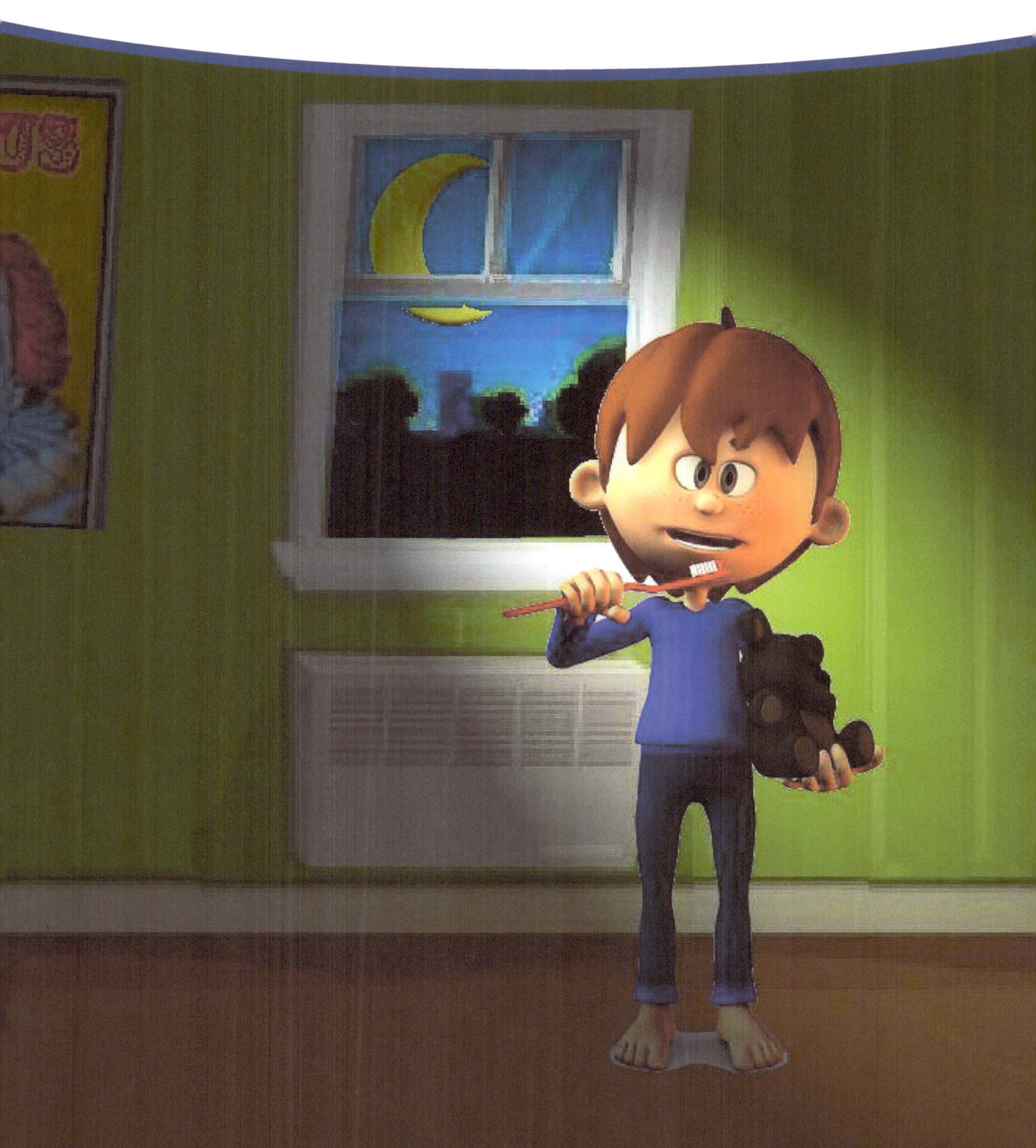

Harry's mother was proud of him too, he really was a big boy now.

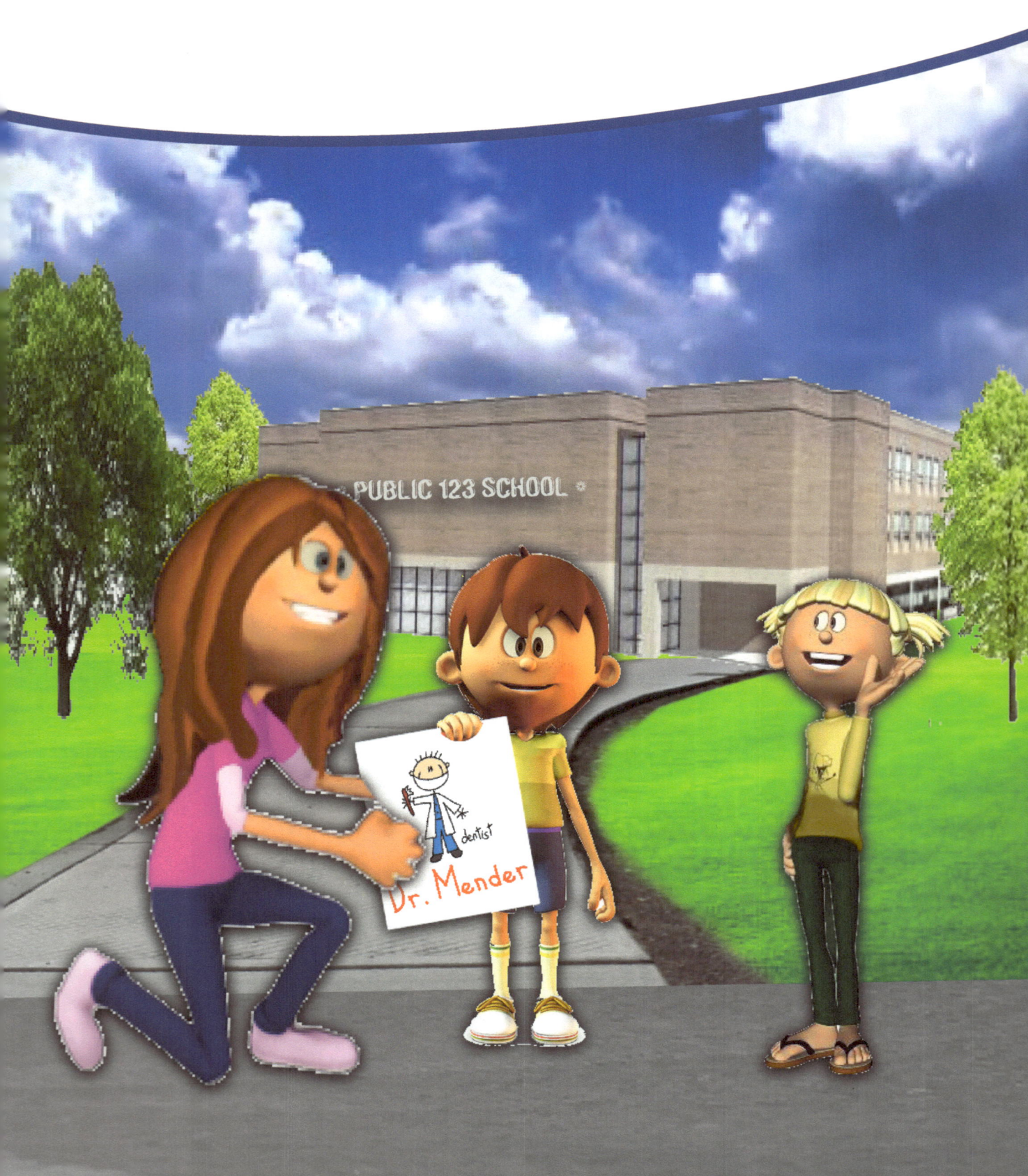

THE END.

ALSO AVAILABLE FROM
the Plaque Pixie Children's book series:

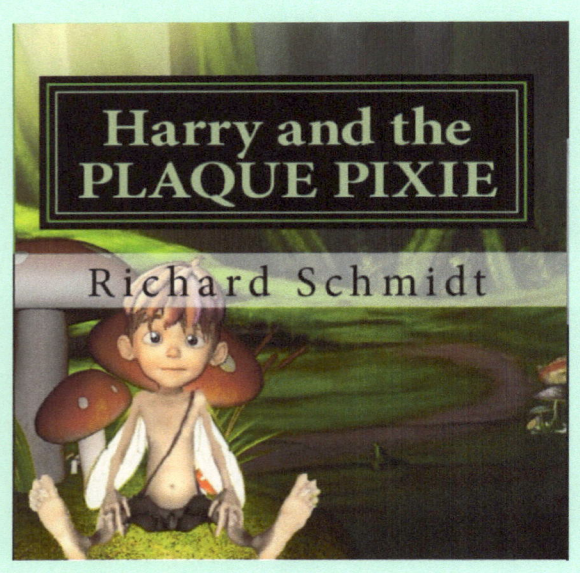

On the morning that the long awaited circus arrives in Harry's town, he gets some unwelcome visitors, the dreaded plaque bugs. Fearing that he will miss the circus, Harry rushes to the dentist for help. Realizing he is in over his head, the dentist calls on the Plaque Pixie to save the day... but will there be time?

FOR MORE INFORMATION VISIT
www.PLAQUEPIXIE.com

www.ingramcontent.com/pod-product-compliance
Lightning Source LLC
Chambersburg PA
CBHW050428180526
45159CB00005B/2455